OSTEOPOROSIS DIET COOKBOOK FOR SENIORS

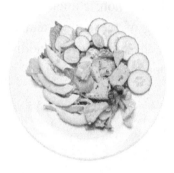

Delicious calcium-rich recipes to naturally promote bone health for older people

Dr. Pamela D. Mathis

DEDICATION

To all those navigating the silent struggles of osteoporosis,

This book is for you, the unsung heroes weaving courage through the delicate dance with fragility and resilience in the shadows of uncertainty. You, dear reader, are the heartbeat of these pages, and your strength echoes in ways words can only strive to express.

To the many souls who've shared stories, fears, and dreams, and to those who endure quietly, this book is a living tribute to your spirit. Beyond the recipes lies a promise of hope, healing, and of the warmth that comes from nourishing both body and soul.

In your journey, you've shown that the human spirit can rise, unyielding in the face of adversity; that love and determination can overcome even the most formidable challenges.

As you explore this cookbook, may it be more than just recipes; may it be a companion on your path to fortified bones, improved health, and a life overflowing with the unbridled joy you so rightfully deserve.

With heartfelt gratitude and boundless hope,

Dr. Pamela D. Mathis

TABLE OF CONTENTS

INTRODUCTION_____7

PART ONE:_____11

Osteoporosis: A Comprehensive Overview: _____ 11

Types of osteoporosis: _____ 11

Symptoms of Osteoporosis:_____ 12

Causes of Osteoporosis: _____ 14

Preventive Measures for Osteoporosis: _____ 15

PART TWO: _____19

The Advantages of an Osteoporosis Diet for Seniors: 19

Foods to consume, limit, and avoid: _____ 23

Complications of osteoporosis if the proper diet is not followed:_____ 28

14-DAY MEAL PLAN _____32

PART THREE: _____37

HEALING BREAKFAST RECIPES:_____ 37

LUNCH RECIPES: _____ 47

DINNER RECIPES: _____ 69

SNACK AND DESSERT RECIPES: _____ 88

JUICE AND SMOOTHIE RECIPES:_____ 95

CONCLUSION_____101

INTRODUCTION

Greetings,

I'm Dr. Pamela D. Mathis, and I'm thrilled to welcome you to the "OSTEOPOROSIS DIET COOKBOOK FOR SENIORS: Delicious calcium-rich recipes to naturally promote bone health for older people." Within these pages, you're not just holding a cookbook; you're cradling a transformative journey toward stronger bones and a healthier, more vibrant life.

Let me share a story close to my heart. I met an extraordinary woman, much like yourself, who had been grappling with the silent adversary— osteoporosis. Her name is Grace and she found herself encumbered by the fear of fractures and the pain that seemed to linger endlessly.

But here's where the magic happens—by embracing the power of the scientifically proven recipes embedded in this cookbook, Grace experienced a remarkable resurgence.

Imagine a life where lifting a grandchild, taking leisurely walks, and dancing at family gatherings become not just memories but a daily reality.

The problem is clear: osteoporosis can cast a daunting shadow on the simplest moments, robbing us of the freedom to move and live without fear. The solution lies within these pages. This cookbook is a compass guiding you towards a path of rejuvenation, offering not just recipes but a lifeline to better bone health.

The dishes you'll discover aren't just delicious; they're a testament to the incredible synergy between taste and health. I crafted this cookbook with decades of expertise, aiming to demystify the journey to bone strength and empower you with the tools to overcome osteoporosis.

So, whether you're seeking a way to alleviate your own struggles or supporting a loved one on this journey, consider this cookbook your ally.

It's time to turn the page on osteoporosis and savor the nourishing recipes that will redefine what it means to age with strength and grace.

Here's to your journey of transformation—one delicious bite at a time.

Warm regards,

Dr. Pamela D. Mathis

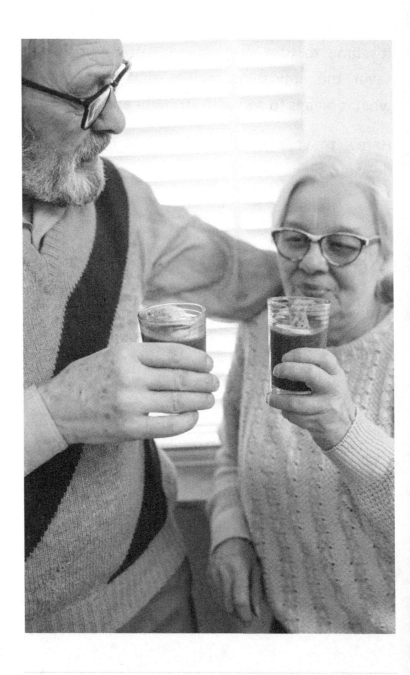

PART ONE:

Osteoporosis: A Comprehensive Overview:

Osteoporosis is a common bone disorder characterized by weakened bones, making them more susceptible to fractures. Often referred to as a "silent disease," it progresses without noticeable symptoms until a fracture occurs. Understanding its types, causes, symptoms, and preventive measures is crucial for maintaining bone health, particularly in aging populations.

Types of osteoporosis:

There are two kinds of osteoporosis:

1. Primary Osteoporosis: This is the most prevalent kind and is more usually connected with ageing and hormonal changes. There are two major types of primary osteoporosis:

I. Osteoporosis after Menopause: It is more common in women after menopause and is caused by a decrease in oestrogen levels, which is important for bone density maintenance.

II. Osteoporosis Due to Age: This kind, which affects both men and women, is associated to the normal ageing process and the steady decrease of bone density over time.

2. Secondary osteoporosis: This is caused by underlying medical disorders or drugs that affect bone health. Secondary osteoporosis can be caused by conditions such as hyperparathyroidism, malabsorption problems, and long-term steroid usage.

Symptoms of Osteoporosis:

Osteoporosis frequently advances gradually, with no noticeable signs, until a fracture occurs. Hip, spine, and wrist fractures are the most frequent osteoporosis-related fractures.

However, there are certain subtle indications that might indicate the existence of osteoporosis, such as:

1. Back Pain: Chronic back pain caused by fractures or the collapse of fragile vertebrae.

2. Height reduction: Osteoporosis can cause a progressive reduction of height over time.

3. Stooped Posture: Also known as "dowager's hump," this is caused by spine curvature as a result of fractures.

4. Bone Fractures: Fractures in the hip, wrist, or spine, in particular, can occur more readily and with less power.

It's important to note that osteoporosis can go undetected for years, so early identification through bone density testing is critical.

Causes of Osteoporosis:

Understanding the root causes of osteoporosis is critical for prevention and therapy. The following are the key variables that contribute to the development of osteoporosis:

1. **Ageing:** As we become older, our bones lose density and become more prone to fractures.

2. **Hormonal Changes:** Hormonal variations, notably oestrogen decline in postmenopausal women, are a substantial risk factor for osteoporosis. A drop in testosterone levels in males can also lead to bone loss.

3. **Family History:** An osteoporosis family history might enhance one's risk.

4. **Dietary Choices:** Bones can be weakened by poor diet, a lack of calcium, and a lack of vitamin D.

5. **Lifestyle Factors:** A sedentary lifestyle, lack of physical activity, smoking, excessive alcohol

intake, and a sedentary lifestyle can all contribute to bone loss.

6. Medical Conditions: Hyperparathyroidism, rheumatoid arthritis, and gastrointestinal issues can all contribute to secondary osteoporosis.

7. Drugs: Long-term use of drugs such as corticosteroids, anticonvulsants, and some cancer therapies can cause bone weakness.

Preventive Measures for Osteoporosis:

The good news is that there are a number of preventative strategies and lifestyle adjustments that can help to minimise the risk of osteoporosis:

1. A Balanced Diet: Make sure your diet is high in calcium and vitamin D, both of which are necessary for bone health. Dairy products, leafy greens, and fortified meals are high in calcium.

2. Regular Exercise: Weight-bearing workouts such as walking, running, and strength training can assist in the development and maintenance of bone density.

3. Changes in Lifestyle: Quit smoking and restrict alcohol use, as both can lead to bone loss.

4. Bone Density Testing: Regular bone density scans can aid in the early detection of osteoporosis, allowing for appropriate intervention.

5. Medication: In some circumstances, healthcare practitioners may offer osteoporosis medication. These should be taken in combination with a change in lifestyle.

6. Fall Prevention: Take actions to lower your chance of falling, such as making sure your house is well-lit, utilizing handrails, and avoiding tripping hazards.

Osteoporosis is a complicated disorder that affects bone health, and understanding its different varieties, causes, symptoms, and preventative actions is critical in dealing with this hidden but serious threat. You may reinforce your bones, minimize the chance of fractures, and live a more active and independent life as you age by adopting a bone-healthy lifestyle and seeking early diagnosis and treatment when necessary. Remember that investing in your bone health is an investment in your entire well-being.

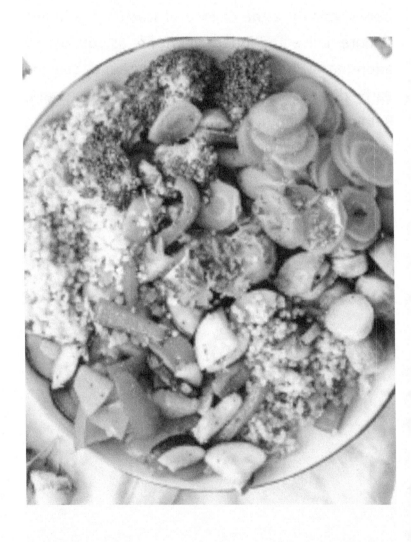

PART TWO:

The Advantages of an Osteoporosis Diet for Seniors:

Following an osteoporosis diet for seniors can provide a number of key advantages for controlling and avoiding this illness. Here are the main benefits:

Improved Bone Health: An osteoporosis diet emphasizes calcium and other important minerals for bone health, such as vitamin D, vitamin K, and magnesium. Consuming these nutrients helps to build bones, reduces the chance of fractures, and slows bone loss, resulting in increased bone density.

Fracture Risk is reduced: Strong bones are less prone to fractures. Seniors may dramatically reduce their chance of devastating fractures, which are especially frequent in osteoporosis, by maintaining optimal bone health with a well-balanced diet.

Muscular Function: A diet high in protein, especially from lean sources, promotes muscular health. Strong muscles contribute to general mobility and can assist elders maintain balance, lowering the risk of fractures from falls.

Improved Joint Health: Fruits and vegetables, for example, include antioxidants and anti-inflammatory substances that can help control joint pain and stiffness, which are frequently connected with osteoporosis.

Independence: Seniors with strong bones and muscles may keep their independence and carry on with their everyday activities without the need for help. This results in a better quality of life and increased self-sufficiency.

Enhanced Nutrient Absorption: Foods that promote greater nutritional absorption, such as those high in vitamin C, are frequently included in an osteoporosis diet. This improves the body's capacity to adequately use important bone-strengthening nutrients.

Heart Health: Many osteoporosis diet components, such as low-sodium options and healthy fats, promote cardiovascular health. Seniors can benefit from improved bone health as well as a lower chance of heart disease.

Weight Control: A well-balanced diet can help elders maintain a healthy weight. Excess body weight puts undue strain on the bones and joints, whereas being underweight increases the chance of fractures. A healthy and stable weight is promoted by an osteoporosis diet.

Medication Dependence might Be Reduced: A well-managed diet might possibly lessen the requirement for osteoporosis drugs. This not only reduces the possibility of negative effects, but also improves general health and well-being.

Slower course of Osteoporosis: Seniors who follow an osteoporosis diet might delay the course of the illness. This implies they will be able to better manage and control the symptoms and problems of osteoporosis.

Better Overall Nutrition: An osteoporosis diet promotes the intake of nutrient-rich foods, which can result in enhanced overall nutrition and well-being. It ensures that seniors get the vitamins and minerals they require for good health.

Lower chance of Falls: Foods strong in protein and calcium, which improve muscular strength and balance, can help seniors maintain their stability and minimize the chance of falling, which is a significant cause of fractures in older persons.

A geriatric osteoporosis diet takes a multifaceted approach to controlling and preventing the illness. It improves not only bone health but also general well-being, independence, and a higher quality of life. Seniors can greatly improve their physical health and lower their risk of osteoporosis-related problems by selecting dietary choices that prioritize necessary nutrients.

Foods to consume, limit, or avoid:

Achieving and maintaining optimal bone and joint health is critical for general health, and it is especially important while dealing with osteoporosis. A well-planned diet can be an effective strategy for controlling this illness. In this article, we'll look at the foods to eat, restrict, and avoid in order to promote healthy bones and joints.

Dairy Products: Dairy products such as milk, yoghurt, and cheese are high in calcium, which is an important building block for bones. To limit your saturated fat consumption, use low-fat or non-fat variants.

Leafy Greens: Kale, broccoli, and collard greens are high in calcium and other critical elements such as vitamin K, which assists in bone mineralization.

Fatty Fish: Salmon, mackerel, and sardines are high in vitamin D and omega-3 fatty acids, which are beneficial to bone health.

Fortified Foods: Many foods, such as fortified cereals and orange juice, include additional calcium and vitamin D. These can be beneficial additions to your diet.

Nuts and Seeds: Almonds, chia seeds, and sesame seeds include calcium, magnesium, and other elements that are essential for bone health.

Lean Proteins: To preserve muscular and bone health, use lean protein sources such as chicken, tofu, and beans.

Whole Grains: Whole grains, such as brown rice and whole wheat bread, include important elements such as magnesium, which aids in bone health.

Fruits: Fruits, such as oranges and berries, include vitamin C, which promotes collagen formation, which is essential for bone and joint health.

Low-Fat Dairy Alternatives: If you are lactose intolerant or prefer non-dairy options, pick calcium- and vitamin D-enriched almond milk, soy milk, or other alternatives.

Foods to limit:

Red Meat: While lean cuts of red meat are high in protein, they should be taken in moderation. Excessive consumption of red meat can create an acidic environment in the body, potentially harming bone health.

Salt: High-sodium diets can cause calcium loss in the urine, which is bad for bone health. Limit your salt consumption by eating fewer processed and packaged meals.

Caffeine: Caffeine use in excess may contribute to calcium loss. Limit your consumption of coffee, tea, and caffeinated beverages.

Soda and Sugary Beverages: Sodas and sugary drinks contain phosphoric acid, which can interfere with calcium absorption. Choose healthier beverages, such as water or herbal teas.

Alcohol: Heavy alcohol use can weaken bones and increase the likelihood of fractures. Drink in moderation if you wish to do so.

Meals to Avoid:

Highly Processed Foods: Processed meals are frequently heavy in salt, sugar, and harmful fats, which can harm general health, especially bone and joint health.

Trans Fats: Trans fats, which are commonly found in processed and fried meals, can cause inflammation and may impair bone density.

Excessive Sweets: Excessive sugar consumption can cause inflammation and impair the body's capacity to absorb calcium.

Highly Acidic Foods: Foods that promote an acidic environment in the body, such as too much meat and certain cereals, might potentially lead to bone deterioration.

Excessive Salty Snacks: Potato chips, pretzels, and other salty snacks can result in high sodium consumption, which can contribute to calcium loss.

A healthy lifestyle, in addition to food choices, is critical for bone and joint health. To increase bone development and preserve muscular strength, engage in weight-bearing exercises such as walking or resistance training. Adequate vitamin D consumption, via sunshine exposure and supplementation if necessary, is also essential, as it aids the body's calcium absorption.

You can successfully treat osteoporosis and create a greater quality of life by making intelligent dietary choices and taking a holistic approach to bone and joint health. Remember that your nutrition is an important part of your road to stronger bones and healthier joints.

Complications of osteoporosis if the proper diet is not followed:

Osteoporosis can lead to a number of major issues if the proper diet and treatment techniques are not followed. These issues can have a substantial influence on a person's overall health and quality of life. Some of the most prevalent problems linked with untreated or poorly managed osteoporosis are as follows:

Fractures: Bone fractures are the most common and acute consequence of osteoporosis. Weakened bones are more prone to fractures, especially in the hip, spine, and wrist. These fractures can occur as a result of mild falls or ordinary activities, resulting in discomfort, impairment, and loss of freedom.

Chronic back discomfort can be caused by osteoporotic fractures, particularly vertebral fractures.

This chronic pain can have a substantial impact on a person's quality of life and make regular tasks difficult.

Fractures and persistent pain can also cause decreased mobility. This restriction on physical activity can cause muscular weakening and loss of balance, raising the risk of falls and subsequent fractures.

Kyphosis (Dowager's Hump): Multiple vertebral fractures can cause the spine to bend forward, resulting in kyphosis (Dowager's Hump). This shift in posture not only has an impact on physical appearance, but it can also lead to back discomfort and respiratory issues.

Hospitalization: Fractures, especially hip fractures, frequently necessitate hospitalization and surgery. Individuals, particularly seniors, may find hospital stays physically and emotionally taxing.

Surgical consequences: Fracture repair surgery carries its own set of risks and consequences, such as infection, blood clots, and anesthesia-related difficulties.

Loss of Independence: Osteoporosis can cause a loss of independence due to discomfort, fractures, and movement limits. Seniors may need help with daily duties, which may be emotionally draining.

Psychological Impact: Osteoporosis-related issues can have a significant psychological impact, including despair, anxiety, and a general sensation of unease. These emotional difficulties are exacerbated by chronic pain, changed body image, and loss of independence.

Reduced Quality of Life: All of the issues discussed above lead to a worse quality of life. Individuals may find it difficult to participate in social events, exercise, or pursue hobbies and interests that they formerly enjoyed.

Increased Healthcare expenses: Managing osteoporosis problems, such as fractures, surgeries, and hospital stays, can result in considerable healthcare expenses, putting a financial strain on people and healthcare systems.

Risk of other Fractures: Once an individual has had an osteoporotic fracture, their risk of other fractures increases. The "fracture cascade" adds to the physical and financial strain.

It should be noted that osteoporosis is frequently preventable and treatable by lifestyle modifications such as a bone-healthy diet, weight-bearing exercise, and appropriate medication therapies. Early identification and treatment can help patients preserve their bone health and general well-being by greatly lowering the chance of problems. As a result, those at risk of osteoporosis must take preventative steps.

14-DAY MEAL PLAN

Day 1:

Breakfast: Greek Yogurt Parfait **(Pg 37)**

Lunch: Salmon and Broccoli Quinoa Bowl **(Pg 47)**

Dinner: Grilled Citrus Salmon **(Pg 69)**

Snack: Roasted Chickpeas **(Pg 90)**

Day 2:

Breakfast: Spinach and Mushroom Omelette **(Pg 38)**

Lunch: Kale and Chickpea Salad **(Pg 48)**

Dinner: Quinoa and Vegetable Stir-Fry **(Pg 70)**

Snack: Cottage Cheese with Pineapple **(Pg 89)**

Day 3:

Breakfast: Chia Seed Pudding **(Pg 39)**

Lunch: Mushroom and Spinach Frittata **(Pg 49)**

Dinner: Baked Lemon Herb Chicken **(Pg 71)**

Snack: Banana Almond Smoothie **(Pg 88)**

Day 4:

Breakfast: Quinoa Breakfast Bowl **(Pg 40)**

Lunch: Turkey and Avocado Wrap **(Pg 50)**

Dinner: Stuffed Bell Peppers with Turkey and Quinoa **(Pg 72)**

Snack: Baked Apple with Cinnamon **(Pg 91)**

Day 5:

Breakfast: Salmon and Avocado Toast **(Pg 41)**

Lunch: Sweet Potato and Lentil Soup **(Pg 51)**

Dinner: Spaghetti Squash with Tomato Basil Sauce **(Pg 73)**

Snack: Chocolate Avocado Mousse **(Pg 92)**

Day 6:

Breakfast: Almond Berry Smoothie **(Pg 42)**

Lunch: Chicken and Quinoa Stuffed Bell Peppers **(Pg 53)**

Dinner: Cauliflower and Broccoli Gratin **(Pg 75)**

Snack: Cucumber and Hummus Bites **(Pg 93)**

Day 7:

Breakfast: Sweet Potato and Kale Hash **(Pg 43)**

Lunch: Tuna and White Bean Salad **(Pg 55)**

Dinner: Lemon Garlic Shrimp with Asparagus **(Pg 76)**

Snack: Yogurt-Dipped Strawberries **(Pg 94)**

Day 8:

Breakfast: Cottage Cheese and Pineapple Bowl **(Pg 44)**

Lunch: Veggie and Hummus Wrap **(Pg 56)**

Dinner: Mushroom and Spinach Stuffed Chicken Breast **(Pg 78)**

Snack: Roasted Chickpeas **(Pg 90)**

Day 9:

Breakfast: Mango and Turmeric Smoothie Bowl **(Pg 45)**

Lunch: Salmon and Asparagus Stir-Fry **(Pg 58)**

Dinner: Eggplant and Tomato Grilled Sandwich **(Pg 79)**

Snack: Baked Apple with Cinnamon **(Pg 91)**

Day 10:

Breakfast: Whole Grain Pancakes with Berries **(Pg 46)**

Lunch: Cauliflower and Chickpea Curry **(Pg 59)**

Dinner: Turkey and Vegetable Skewers **(Pg 81)**

Snack: Chocolate Avocado Mousse **(Pg 92)**

Day 11:

Breakfast: Greek Yogurt Parfait **(Pg 37)**

Lunch: Shrimp and Broccoli Stir-Fry **(Pg 61)**

Dinner: Chickpea and Spinach Curry **(Pg 82)**

Snack: Banana Almond Smoothie **(Pg 88)**

Day 12:

Breakfast: Spinach and Mushroom Omelette **(Pg 38)**

Lunch: Baked Eggplant Parmesan **(Pg 62)**

Dinner: Salmon and Spinach Stuffed Sweet Potatoes **(Pg 84)**

Snack: Yogurt-Dipped Strawberries **(Pg 94)**

Day 13:

Breakfast: Chia Seed Pudding **(Pg 39)**

Lunch: Chickpea and Vegetable Curry **(Pg 64)**

Dinner: Quinoa and Vegetable Stir-Fry **(Pg 85)**

Snack: Roasted Chickpeas **(Pg 90)**

Day 14:

Breakfast: Quinoa Breakfast Bowl **(Pg 40)**

Lunch: Stuffed Acorn Squash **(Pg 66)**

Dinner: Baked Chicken with Brussels Sprouts **(Pg 86)**

Snack: Cucumber and Hummus Bites **(Pg 93)**

Enjoy these flavorful and nourishing meals!

PART THREE:

HEALING BREAKFAST RECIPES:

1. Greek Yogurt Parfait:

Ingredients:

- ❖ 1 cup Greek yogurt
- ❖ 1/2 cup fresh berries (blueberries, strawberries)
- ❖ 1 tablespoon chia seeds
- ❖ 1 tablespoon chopped nuts (almonds, walnuts)

Preparation:

1. In a glass or bowl, layer Greek yogurt, berries, chia seeds, and nuts.
2. Repeat layers.

Servings: 1

Nutritional Value: Calcium: 350mg, Vitamin D: 15 IU, Carbs: 20g, Fat: 15g

Cooking Time: 5 minutes

2. Spinach and Mushroom Omelette:

Ingredients:

- ❖ 2 eggs
- ❖ 1/2 cup spinach, chopped
- ❖ 1/4 cup mushrooms, sliced
- ❖ 1 tablespoon feta cheese

Preparation:

1. Whisk eggs and pour into a hot, non-stick pan.
2. Add spinach, mushrooms, and feta. Fold the omelette.

Servings: 1

Nutritional Value:

- ❖ Calcium: 200mg
- ❖ Vitamin D: 80 IU
- ❖ Carbs: 4g
- ❖ Fat: 12g

Cooking Time: 10 minutes

3. Chia Seed Pudding:

Ingredients:

- ❖ 2 tablespoons chia seeds
- ❖ 1 cup unsweetened almond milk
- ❖ 1/2 teaspoon vanilla extract
- ❖ 1/4 cup sliced kiwi

Preparation:

1. Mix chia seeds, almond milk, and vanilla. Refrigerate for at least 2 hours.
2. Top with sliced kiwi before serving.

Servings: 1

Nutritional Value:

- ❖ Calcium: 300mg
- ❖ Vitamin D: 40 IU
- ❖ Carbs: 15g
- ❖ Fat: 10g

Cooking Time: 2 hours (including refrigeration)

4. Quinoa Breakfast Bowl:

Ingredients:

- ❖ 1/2 cup cooked quinoa
- ❖ 1/4 cup sliced peaches
- ❖ 1 tablespoon pumpkin seeds
- ❖ Drizzle of honey

Preparation:

1. Combine cooked quinoa, sliced peaches, and pumpkin seeds.
2. Drizzle with honey.

Servings: 1

Nutritional Value:

- ❖ Calcium: 150mg
- ❖ Vitamin D: 30 IU
- ❖ Carbs: 30g
- ❖ Fat: 5g

Cooking Time: 15 minutes

5. Salmon and Avocado Toast:

Ingredients:

- ❖ 1 slice whole-grain bread
- ❖ 2 oz smoked salmon
- ❖ 1/2 avocado, sliced
- ❖ 1 teaspoon lemon juice

Preparation:

1. Toast the bread and top with smoked salmon and avocado slices.
2. Drizzle with lemon juice.

Servings: 1

Nutritional Value:

- ❖ Calcium: 100mg
- ❖ Vitamin D: 150 IU
- ❖ Carbs: 15g
- ❖ Fat: 10g

Cooking Time: 5 minutes

6. Almond Berry Smoothie:

Ingredients:

- ❖ 1 cup almond milk
- ❖ 1/2 cup mixed berries (strawberries, raspberries, blueberries)
- ❖ 1 tablespoon almond butter
- ❖ 1 scoop collagen powder (optional)

Preparation:

1. Blend almond milk, mixed berries, almond butter, and collagen powder until smooth.

Servings: 1

Nutritional Value:

- ❖ Calcium: 250mg
- ❖ Vitamin D: 50 IU
- ❖ Carbs: 20g
- ❖ Fat: 12g

Cooking Time: 5 minutes

7. Sweet Potato and Kale Hash:

Ingredients:

- ❖ 1/2 cup sweet potatoes, diced
- ❖ 1/2 cup kale, chopped
- ❖ 1 egg
- ❖ 1 teaspoon olive oil

Preparation:

1. Sauté sweet potatoes and kale in olive oil until cooked.
2. Top with a fried egg.

Servings: 1

Nutritional Value:

- ❖ Calcium: 180mg
- ❖ Vitamin D: 60 IU
- ❖ Carbs: 20g
- ❖ Fat: 10g

Cooking Time: 15 minutes

8. Cottage Cheese and Pineapple Bowl:

Ingredients:

- ❖ 1/2 cup low-fat cottage cheese
- ❖ 1/2 cup fresh pineapple chunks
- ❖ 1 tablespoon sunflower seeds
- ❖ Drizzle of honey

Preparation:

1. Mix cottage cheese, pineapple chunks, and sunflower seeds.
2. Drizzle with honey before serving.

Servings: 1

Nutritional Value:

- ❖ Calcium: 250mg
- ❖ Vitamin D: 40 IU
- ❖ Carbs: 20g
- ❖ Fat: 8g

Cooking Time: 5 minutes

9. Mango and Turmeric Smoothie Bowl:

Ingredients:

- ❖ 1 cup mango chunks (frozen or fresh)
- ❖ 1/2 teaspoon turmeric powder
- ❖ 1/2 cup unsweetened coconut milk
- ❖ **Toppings:** sliced banana, shredded coconut

Preparation:

1. Blend mango, turmeric, and coconut milk until smooth.
2. Top with sliced banana and shredded coconut.

Servings: 1

Nutritional Value:

- ❖ Calcium: 150mg
- ❖ Vitamin D: 30 IU
- ❖ Carbs: 25g
- ❖ Fat: 7g

Cooking Time: 5 minutes

10. Whole Grain Pancakes with Berries:

Ingredients:

- ❖ 1/2 cup whole grain pancake mix
- ❖ 1/2 cup mixed berries (blueberries, strawberries)
- ❖ 1 tablespoon flaxseeds
- ❖ Maple syrup (optional)

Preparation:

1. Prepare pancakes according to the mix instructions.
2. Top with mixed berries and flaxseeds. Add maple syrup if desired.

Servings: 1

Nutritional Value:

- ❖ Calcium: 200mg
- ❖ Vitamin D: 20 IU
- ❖ Carbs: 30g
- ❖ Fat: 5g

Cooking Time: 15 minutes

LUNCH RECIPES:

1. Salmon and Broccoli Quinoa Bowl:

Ingredients:

- ❖ 1/2 cup cooked quinoa
- ❖ 4 oz grilled salmon
- ❖ 1 cup steamed broccoli
- ❖ 1 tablespoon olive oil

Preparation:

1. Cook quinoa according to package instructions.
2. Grill salmon and steam broccoli.
3. Arrange quinoa, salmon, and broccoli in a bowl.
4. Drizzle with olive oil.

Servings: 1

Nutritional Value: Calcium: 250mg, Vitamin D: 150 IU, Carbs: 20g, Fat: 15g

Cooking Time: 15 minutes

2. Kale and Chickpea Salad:

Ingredients:

- ❖ 2 cups kale, chopped
- ❖ 1/2 cup chickpeas, drained and rinsed
- ❖ 1/4 cup feta cheese, crumbled
- ❖ 1/4 cup cherry tomatoes, halved
- ❖ 1 tablespoon balsamic vinaigrette

Preparation:

1. In a large bowl, combine chopped kale, chickpeas, feta cheese, and cherry tomatoes.
2. Drizzle with balsamic vinaigrette and toss until well coated.
3. Serve immediately.

Servings: 1

Nutritional Value: Calcium: 200mg, Vitamin D: 80 IU, Carbs: 25g, Fat: 10g

Preparation Time: 10 minutes

3. Mushroom and Spinach Frittata:

Ingredients:

- ❖ 2 eggs
- ❖ 1/2 cup mushrooms, sliced
- ❖ 1 cup spinach, chopped
- ❖ 1/4 cup Parmesan cheese, grated
- ❖ Salt and pepper to taste

Preparation:

1. Preheat the oven to 375°F (190°C).
2. In a bowl, whisk eggs and season with salt and pepper.
3. In an oven-safe skillet, sauté mushrooms until softened. Add spinach and cook until wilted.
4. Pour the whisked eggs over the vegetables in the skillet.
5. Sprinkle Parmesan cheese on top.
6. Bake in the preheated oven for 15-20 minutes or until the frittata is set.
7. Slice and serve.

Servings: 1

Nutritional Value: Calcium: 180mg, Vitamin D: 60 IU, Carbs: 4g, Fat: 12g

Cooking Time: 25 minutes

4. Turkey and Avocado Wrap:

Ingredients:

- ❖ 1 whole-grain tortilla
- ❖ 3 oz sliced turkey
- ❖ 1/2 avocado, sliced
- ❖ 1/2 cup mixed greens
- ❖ Mustard (optional)

Preparation:

1. Lay the whole-grain tortilla flat on a clean surface.
2. Layer the turkey, avocado slices, and mixed greens on the tortilla.
3. Optionally, add mustard for extra flavor.
4. Roll the tortilla tightly into a wrap.
5. Slice and serve.

Servings: 1

Nutritional Value: Calcium: 150mg, Vitamin D: 40 IU, Carbs: 30g, Fat: 10g

Preparation Time: 10 minutes

5. Sweet Potato and Lentil Soup:

Ingredients:

- ❖ 1 cup sweet potatoes, diced
- ❖ 1/2 cup lentils, rinsed and drained
- ❖ 1/2 cup carrots, chopped
- ❖ 1/2 cup celery, chopped
- ❖ 1/2 onion, diced
- ❖ 2 cloves garlic, minced
- ❖ 4 cups vegetable broth
- ❖ 1 teaspoon cumin
- ❖ 1/2 teaspoon paprika
- ❖ Salt and pepper to taste
- ❖ Fresh parsley for garnish

Preparation:

1. In a large pot, sauté onions and garlic until fragrant.
2. Add sweet potatoes, lentils, carrots, and celery to the pot.
3. Pour in vegetable broth and season with cumin, paprika, salt, and pepper.
4. Bring the soup to a boil, then reduce the heat and simmer for 20-25 minutes or until lentils are tender.
5. Garnish with fresh parsley before serving.

Servings: 4

Nutritional Value:

- ❖ Calcium: 200mg
- ❖ Vitamin D: 50 IU
- ❖ Carbs: 35g
- ❖ Fat: 1g

Cooking Time: 30 minutes

6. Chicken and Quinoa Stuffed Bell Peppers:

Ingredients:

- ❖ 2 bell peppers, halved and seeds removed
- ❖ 1/2 cup quinoa, cooked
- ❖ 1/2 cup cooked chicken breast, shredded
- ❖ 1/4 cup black beans, drained and rinsed
- ❖ 1/4 cup corn kernels
- ❖ 1/4 cup diced tomatoes
- ❖ 1/4 cup shredded cheddar cheese
- ❖ 1 teaspoon cumin
- ❖ 1/2 teaspoon chili powder
- ❖ Salt and pepper to taste

Preparation:

1. Preheat the oven to 375°F (190°C).
2. In a bowl, combine cooked quinoa, shredded chicken, black beans, corn, diced tomatoes, cumin, chili powder, salt, and pepper.

3. Stuff each bell pepper half with the quinoa mixture.
4. Top with shredded cheddar cheese.
5. Place the stuffed peppers in a baking dish and bake for 20-25 minutes or until the peppers are tender.
6. Serve warm.

Servings: 2

Nutritional Value:

- ❖ Calcium: 150mg
- ❖ Vitamin D: 40 IU
- ❖ Carbs: 30g
- ❖ Fat: 7g

Cooking Time: 30 minutes

7. Tuna and White Bean Salad:

Ingredients:

- ❖ 1 can (5 oz) tuna, drained
- ❖ 1 cup white beans, cooked
- ❖ 1/2 cucumber, diced
- ❖ 1/4 red onion, finely chopped
- ❖ 1/4 cup Kalamata olives, sliced
- ❖ 2 tablespoons olive oil
- ❖ 1 tablespoon red wine vinegar
- ❖ 1 teaspoon Dijon mustard
- ❖ Salt and pepper to taste
- ❖ Fresh parsley for garnish

Preparation:

1. In a large bowl, combine tuna, white beans, cucumber, red onion, and olives.
2. In a small bowl, whisk together olive oil, red wine vinegar, Dijon mustard, salt, and pepper.
3. Pour the dressing over the salad and toss to coat.

4. Garnish with fresh parsley before serving.

Servings: 2

Nutritional Value:

- ❖ Calcium: 200mg
- ❖ Vitamin D: 80 IU
- ❖ Carbs: 25g
- ❖ Fat: 15g

Preparation Time: 15 minutes

8. Veggie and Hummus Wrap:

Ingredients:

- ❖ 1 whole-grain tortilla
- ❖ 1/4 cup hummus
- ❖ 1/2 cup mixed vegetables (bell peppers, cucumbers, carrots), thinly sliced
- ❖ 1/4 cup baby spinach leaves
- ❖ 1 tablespoon feta cheese, crumbled

Preparation:

1. Spread hummus evenly over the whole-grain tortilla.
2. Layer the mixed vegetables, baby spinach, and crumbled feta on one side of the tortilla.
3. Roll the tortilla tightly into a wrap.
4. Slice and serve.

Servings: 1

Nutritional Value:

❖ Calcium: 150mg
❖ Vitamin D: 40 IU
❖ Carbs: 30g
❖ Fat: 8g

Preparation Time: 10 minutes

9. Salmon and Asparagus Stir-Fry:

Ingredients:

- ❖ 4 oz salmon fillet, cut into cubes
- ❖ 1 cup asparagus, chopped
- ❖ 1/2 cup bell peppers, sliced
- ❖ 1/4 cup soy sauce (low-sodium)
- ❖ 1 tablespoon olive oil
- ❖ 1 tablespoon ginger, minced
- ❖ 2 cloves garlic, minced
- ❖ 1 teaspoon sesame oil
- ❖ Sesame seeds for garnish

Preparation:

1. Heat olive oil in a wok or skillet over medium-high heat.
2. Add ginger and garlic, sauté until fragrant.
3. Add salmon cubes and cook until browned.
4. Add asparagus and bell peppers, stir-fry until vegetables are tender-crisp.

5. Pour in soy sauce and sesame oil, toss until well combined.
6. Garnish with sesame seeds before serving.

Servings: 1

Nutritional Value:

- ❖ Calcium: 250mg
- ❖ Vitamin D: 150 IU
- ❖ Carbs: 15g
- ❖ Fat: 15g

Cooking Time: 15 minutes

10. Cauliflower and Chickpea Curry:

Ingredients:

- ❖ 1 cup cauliflower florets
- ❖ 1/2 cup chickpeas, drained and rinsed
- ❖ 1/2 cup tomatoes, diced
- ❖ 1/4 cup onion, chopped

- ❖ 2 tablespoons curry powder
- ❖ 1 tablespoon coconut oil
- ❖ 1/2 cup coconut milk (light)
- ❖ Fresh cilantro for garnish

Preparation:

1. In a pan, heat coconut oil over medium heat.
2. Add onions and sauté until translucent.
3. Add cauliflower, chickpeas, tomatoes, and curry powder. Cook for 5 minutes.
4. Pour in coconut milk, cover, and simmer for an additional 10 minutes or until cauliflower is tender.
5. Garnish with fresh cilantro before serving.

Servings: 2

Nutritional Value:

- ❖ Calcium: 150mg
- ❖ Vitamin D: 40 IU
- ❖ Carbs: 20g
- ❖ Fat: 10g

Cooking Time: 20 minutes

11. Shrimp and Broccoli Stir-Fry:

Ingredients:

- ❖ 6 oz shrimp, peeled and deveined
- ❖ 2 cups broccoli florets
- ❖ 1/2 cup snap peas
- ❖ 1 tablespoon soy sauce (low-sodium)
- ❖ 1 tablespoon hoisin sauce
- ❖ 1 tablespoon vegetable oil
- ❖ 1 teaspoon sesame seeds for garnish

Preparation:

1. In a wok, heat vegetable oil and stir-fry shrimp until pink.
2. Add broccoli and snap peas, continue stir-frying until vegetables are tender-crisp.
3. Pour in soy sauce and hoisin sauce, toss until well coated.
4. Garnish with sesame seeds before serving.

Servings: 2

Nutritional Value: Calcium: 120mg, Vitamin D: 80 IU, Carbs: 15g, Fat: 10g

Cooking Time: 20 minutes

12. Baked Eggplant Parmesan:

Ingredients:

- ❖ 1 large eggplant, sliced
- ❖ 1 cup marinara sauce (low-sugar)
- ❖ 1 cup mozzarella cheese, shredded
- ❖ 1/2 cup Parmesan cheese, grated
- ❖ 2 tablespoons olive oil
- ❖ Fresh basil for garnish

Preparation:

1. Preheat the oven to 375°F (190°C).
2. Brush eggplant slices with olive oil and bake until golden.
3. In a baking dish, layer eggplant, marinara sauce, and cheeses.
4. Repeat layers and bake until cheese is melted and bubbly.
5. Garnish with fresh basil before serving.

Servings: 3

Nutritional Value: Calcium: 180mg, Vitamin D: 120 IU, Carbs: 15g, Fat: 10g

Cooking Time: 45 minutes

13. Spinach and Feta Stuffed Chicken Breast:

Ingredients:

- ❖ 2 boneless, skinless chicken breasts
- ❖ 1 cup fresh spinach, chopped
- ❖ 1/4 cup feta cheese, crumbled
- ❖ 1 teaspoon garlic powder
- ❖ Salt and pepper to taste
- ❖ 1 tablespoon olive oil

Preparation:

1. Preheat the oven to 400°F (200°C).
2. Season chicken breasts with garlic powder, salt, and pepper.
3. In a bowl, mix chopped spinach and feta.
4. Cut a pocket into each chicken breast and stuff with the spinach and feta mixture.
5. Drizzle with olive oil and bake until chicken is cooked through.

Servings: 2

Nutritional Value: Calcium: 120mg, Vitamin D: 100 IU, Carbs: 2g, Fat: 8g

Cooking Time: 30 minutes

14. Chickpea and Vegetable Curry:

Ingredients:

- ❖ 1 can (15 oz) chickpeas, drained and rinsed
- ❖ 1 cup cauliflower florets
- ❖ 1/2 cup carrots, diced
- ❖ 1/2 cup peas
- ❖ 1/2 cup bell peppers, sliced
- ❖ 1/2 cup tomatoes, diced
- ❖ 1 onion, finely chopped
- ❖ 2 cloves garlic, minced
- ❖ 1 tablespoon curry powder
- ❖ 1 tablespoon coconut oil
- ❖ 1/2 cup coconut milk (light)
- ❖ Fresh cilantro for garnish

Preparation:

1. In a pot, sauté onions and garlic in coconut oil until translucent.
2. Add curry powder and cook until fragrant.
3. Add chickpeas, cauliflower, carrots, peas, bell peppers, and tomatoes. Stir to coat.
4. Pour in coconut milk, cover, and simmer until vegetables are tender.
5. Garnish with fresh cilantro before serving.

Servings: 3

Nutritional Value: Calcium: 100mg, Vitamin D: 80 IU, Carbs: 35g, Fat: 10g

Cooking Time: 25 minutes

15. Stuffed Acorn Squash:

Ingredients:

- ❖ 2 acorn squashes, halved and seeds removed
- ❖ 1 cup quinoa, cooked
- ❖ 1/2 cup dried cranberries
- ❖ 1/4 cup pecans, chopped
- ❖ 1 tablespoon maple syrup
- ❖ 1 tablespoon olive oil
- ❖ Cinnamon for sprinkling

Preparation:

1. Preheat the oven to 375°F (190°C).
2. Roast acorn squashes until tender.
3. In a bowl, mix cooked quinoa, dried cranberries, pecans, maple syrup, and olive oil.
4. Stuff each acorn squash half with the quinoa mixture.
5. Sprinkle with cinnamon before serving.

Servings: 4

Nutritional Value: Calcium: 120mg, Vitamin D: 50 IU, Carbs: 30g, Fat: 8g

Cooking Time: 45 minutes

16. Lemon Garlic Shrimp with Zucchini Noodles:

Ingredients:

- ❖ 6 oz shrimp, peeled and deveined
- ❖ 2 zucchinis, spiralized
- ❖ 2 tablespoons olive oil
- ❖ 2 cloves garlic, minced
- ❖ 1 tablespoon lemon juice
- ❖ Fresh parsley for garnish
- ❖ Salt and pepper to taste

Preparation:

1. In a pan, heat olive oil and sauté garlic until fragrant.
2. Add shrimp and cook until pink.

3. Toss in spiralized zucchini and cook until noodles are tender.
4. Drizzle with lemon juice and season with salt and pepper.
5. Garnish with fresh parsley before serving.

Servings: 2

Nutritional Value:

- ❖ Calcium: 80mg
- ❖ Vitamin D: 100 IU
- ❖ Carbs: 10g

Fat: 8g

DINNER RECIPES:

1. Grilled Citrus Salmon:

Ingredients:

- ❖ 6 oz salmon fillet
- ❖ 1 tablespoon olive oil
- ❖ 1 tablespoon fresh lemon juice
- ❖ 1 tablespoon fresh orange juice
- ❖ 1 teaspoon lemon zest
- ❖ 1 teaspoon honey
- ❖ Salt and pepper to taste

Preparation:

1. Preheat the grill.
2. In a bowl, mix olive oil, lemon juice, orange juice, lemon zest, honey, salt, and pepper.
3. Brush the salmon with the citrus mixture.
4. Grill the salmon for 4-5 minutes per side or until cooked through.

Servings: 1

Nutritional Value: Calcium: 150mg, Vitamin D: 100 IU, Carbs: 5g, Fat: 10g

Cooking Time: 10 minutes

2. Quinoa and Vegetable Stir-Fry:

Ingredients:

- ❖ 1/2 cup cooked quinoa
- ❖ 1 cup mixed vegetables (broccoli, bell peppers, carrots), chopped
- ❖ 2 tablespoons low-sodium soy sauce
- ❖ 1 tablespoon olive oil
- ❖ 1 teaspoon ginger, minced
- ❖ 1 clove garlic, minced

Preparation:

1. In a wok or skillet, heat olive oil over medium-high heat.
2. Add ginger and garlic, sauté until fragrant.
3. Add mixed vegetables and stir-fry for 3-4 minutes.
4. Add cooked quinoa and soy sauce, toss until well combined.

Servings: 1

Nutritional Value: Calcium: 100mg, Vitamin D: 80 IU, Carbs: 30g, Fat: 7g

Cooking Time: 15 minutes

3. Baked Lemon Herb Chicken:

Ingredients:

- ❖ 6 oz chicken breast
- ❖ 1 tablespoon olive oil
- ❖ 1 tablespoon fresh lemon juice
- ❖ 1 teaspoon dried thyme
- ❖ 1 teaspoon dried rosemary
- ❖ Salt and pepper to taste

Preparation:

1. Preheat the oven to 375°F (190°C).
2. In a small bowl, mix olive oil, lemon juice, thyme, rosemary, salt, and pepper.
3. Place the chicken breast in a baking dish and brush with the lemon herb mixture.
4. Bake for 25-30 minutes or until the chicken is cooked through.

Servings: 1

Nutritional Value: Calcium: 50mg, Vitamin D: 120 IU, Carbs: 1g, Fat: 8g

Cooking Time: 30 minutes

4. Stuffed Bell Peppers with Turkey and Quinoa:

Ingredients:

- ❖ 2 bell peppers, halved and seeds removed
- ❖ 1/2 cup cooked quinoa
- ❖ 4 oz lean ground turkey
- ❖ 1/4 cup black beans, drained and rinsed
- ❖ 1/4 cup corn kernels
- ❖ 1/4 cup diced tomatoes
- ❖ 1 teaspoon cumin
- ❖ 1/2 teaspoon chili powder
- ❖ Salt and pepper to taste

Preparation:

1. Preheat the oven to 375°F (190°C).
2. In a skillet, cook ground turkey until browned. Add cumin, chili powder, salt, and pepper.
3. In a bowl, mix cooked quinoa, black beans, corn, diced tomatoes, and cooked turkey.

4. Stuff each bell pepper half with the quinoa mixture.
5. Bake for 20-25 minutes or until the peppers are tender.

Servings: 2

Nutritional Value: Calcium: 100mg, Vitamin D: 60 IU, Carbs: 20g, Fat: 5g

Cooking Time: 30 minutes

5. Spaghetti Squash with Tomato Basil Sauce:

Ingredients:

- ❖ 1 small spaghetti squash
- ❖ 1 cup cherry tomatoes, halved
- ❖ 2 cloves garlic, minced
- ❖ 1 tablespoon olive oil
- ❖ 1/4 cup fresh basil, chopped
- ❖ Salt and pepper to taste

Preparation:

1. Preheat the oven to 375°F (190°C).
2. Cut the spaghetti squash in half lengthwise and remove the seeds.
3. Place the squash, cut side down, on a baking sheet. Bake for 30-40 minutes or until tender.
4. In a skillet, heat olive oil and sauté garlic until fragrant. Add cherry tomatoes, basil, salt, and pepper.
5. Scrape the spaghetti squash with a fork to create "noodles" and toss with the tomato basil sauce.

Servings: 2

Nutritional Value:

- ❖ Calcium: 80mg
- ❖ Vitamin D: 40 IU
- ❖ Carbs: 15g
- ❖ Fat: 5g

Cooking Time: 40 minutes

6. Cauliflower and Broccoli Gratin:

Ingredients:

- ❖ 1 cup cauliflower florets
- ❖ 1 cup broccoli florets
- ❖ 1/2 cup low-fat Greek yogurt
- ❖ 1/4 cup Parmesan cheese, grated
- ❖ 1/4 cup mozzarella cheese, shredded
- ❖ 1 clove garlic, minced
- ❖ 1 teaspoon Dijon mustard
- ❖ Salt and pepper to taste

Preparation:

1. Preheat the oven to 375°F (190°C).
2. Steam cauliflower and broccoli until slightly tender.
3. In a bowl, mix Greek yogurt, Parmesan cheese, mozzarella cheese, garlic, Dijon mustard, salt, and pepper.
4. Combine the steamed cauliflower and broccoli with the yogurt mixture.

5. Transfer to a baking dish and bake for 20-25 minutes or until bubbly and golden.

Servings: 2

Nutritional Value:

- ❖ Calcium: 150mg
- ❖ Vitamin D: 60 IU
- ❖ Carbs: 10g
- ❖ Fat: 8g

Cooking Time: 25 minutes

7. Lemon Garlic Shrimp with Asparagus:

Ingredients:

- ❖ 8 oz shrimp, peeled and deveined
- ❖ 1 bunch asparagus, trimmed
- ❖ 2 tablespoons olive oil
- ❖ 2 cloves garlic, minced
- ❖ 1 tablespoon fresh lemon juice
- ❖ 1 teaspoon lemon zest
- ❖ Salt and pepper to taste

Preparation:

1. In a skillet, heat olive oil over medium-high heat.
2. Add shrimp and asparagus, sauté until shrimp are pink and asparagus is tender.
3. Add garlic, lemon juice, lemon zest, salt, and pepper. Cook for an additional 2 minutes.

Servings: 1

Nutritional Value:

- ❖ Calcium: 100mg
- ❖ Vitamin D: 80 IU
- ❖ Carbs: 5g
- ❖ Fat: 10g

Cooking Time: 15 minutes

8. Mushroom and Spinach Stuffed Chicken Breast:

Ingredients:

- ❖ 6 oz chicken breast
- ❖ 1/2 cup mushrooms, chopped
- ❖ 1 cup spinach, chopped
- ❖ 2 tablespoons feta cheese, crumbled
- ❖ 1 clove garlic, minced
- ❖ 1 tablespoon olive oil
- ❖ Salt and pepper to taste

Preparation:

1. Preheat the oven to 375°F (190°C).
2. In a skillet, heat olive oil over medium heat. Add mushrooms and garlic, sauté until mushrooms release their moisture.
3. Add spinach and cook until wilted. Remove from heat and stir in feta cheese.
4. Slice a pocket in the chicken breast and stuff with the mushroom and spinach mixture.

5. Bake for 25-30 minutes or until the chicken is cooked through.

Servings: 1

Nutritional Value: Calcium: 120mg, Vitamin D: 90 IU, Carbs: 3g, Fat: 12g

Cooking Time: 30 minutes

9. Eggplant and Tomato Grilled Sandwich:

Ingredients:

- ❖ 1/2 medium eggplant, sliced
- ❖ 1 large tomato, sliced
- ❖ 2 slices whole-grain bread
- ❖ 1 tablespoon pesto sauce
- ❖ 1 tablespoon olive oil
- ❖ Salt and pepper to taste

Preparation:

1. Preheat a grill pan or outdoor grill.

2. Brush eggplant slices with olive oil and season with salt and pepper.
3. Grill eggplant slices for 3-4 minutes per side.
4. Spread pesto sauce on one side of each bread slice.
5. Assemble the sandwich with grilled eggplant and tomato slices.
6. Grill the sandwich for 2-3 minutes on each side or until bread is toasted.

Servings: 1

Nutritional Value:

- ❖ Calcium: 80mg
- ❖ Vitamin D: 60 IU
- ❖ Carbs: 30g
- ❖ Fat: 10g

Cooking Time: 10 minutes

10. Turkey and Vegetable Skewers:

Ingredients:

- ❖ 6 oz turkey breast, cut into cubes
- ❖ 1 zucchini, sliced
- ❖ 1 red bell pepper, cut into chunks
- ❖ 1 red onion, cut into chunks
- ❖ 1 tablespoon olive oil
- ❖ 1 teaspoon Italian seasoning
- ❖ Salt and pepper to taste

Preparation:

1. Preheat a grill or grill pan.
2. In a bowl, toss turkey, zucchini, red bell pepper, and red onion with olive oil, Italian seasoning, salt, and pepper.
3. Thread the turkey and vegetables onto skewers.
4. Grill for 10-12 minutes, turning occasionally, until turkey is cooked through and vegetables are tender.

Servings: 1

Nutritional Value: Calcium: 100mg, Vitamin D: 70 IU, Carbs: 10g, Fat: 8g

Cooking Time: 15 minutes

11. Chickpea and Spinach Curry:

Ingredients:

- ❖ 1 can (15 oz) chickpeas, drained and rinsed
- ❖ 2 cups fresh spinach
- ❖ 1/2 cup tomatoes, diced
- ❖ 1/4 cup onion, chopped
- ❖ 2 cloves garlic, minced
- ❖ 1 tablespoon curry powder
- ❖ 1 tablespoon coconut oil
- ❖ 1/2 cup coconut milk (light)
- ❖ Salt and pepper to taste
- ❖ Fresh cilantro for garnish

Preparation:

1. In a pan, heat coconut oil over medium heat.
2. Add onions and sauté until translucent.
3. Add garlic, tomatoes, and curry powder. Cook for 2-3 minutes.
4. Stir in chickpeas and coconut milk. Simmer for 10 minutes.
5. Add fresh spinach and cook until wilted.
6. Season with salt and pepper. Garnish with fresh cilantro before serving.

Servings: 2

Nutritional Value:

- ❖ Calcium: 120mg
- ❖ Vitamin D: 50 IU
- ❖ Carbs: 30g
- ❖ Fat: 10g

Cooking Time: 20 minutes

12. Salmon and Spinach Stuffed Sweet Potatoes:

Ingredients:

- ❖ 2 medium sweet potatoes
- ❖ 6 oz salmon fillet
- ❖ 1 cup fresh spinach
- ❖ 1 tablespoon olive oil
- ❖ Salt and pepper to taste

Preparation:

1. Preheat the oven to 400°F (200°C).
2. Roast sweet potatoes until tender.
3. In a pan, sauté spinach in olive oil until wilted.
4. Grill or bake salmon until cooked.
5. Slice sweet potatoes, stuff with spinach, and top with salmon.

Servings: 2   **Cooking Time:** 40 minutes

Nutritional Value: Calcium: 150mg, Vitamin D: 250 IU, Carbs: 30g, Fat: 10g

13. Quinoa and Vegetable Stir-Fry:

Ingredients:

- ❖ 1/2 cup quinoa
- ❖ 1 cup mixed vegetables (broccoli, bell peppers, carrots)
- ❖ 4 oz tofu, cubed
- ❖ 2 tablespoons soy sauce (low-sodium)
- ❖ 1 tablespoon sesame oil
- ❖ 1 teaspoon ginger, minced

Preparation:

1. Cook quinoa according to package instructions.
2. In a wok, stir-fry mixed vegetables and tofu in sesame oil.
3. Add cooked quinoa and soy sauce. Stir until well combined.
4. Garnish with minced ginger before serving.

Servings: 2

Nutritional Value: Calcium: 120mg, Vitamin D: 100 IU, Carbs: 35g, Fat: 15g

Cooking Time: 25 minutes

14. Baked Chicken with Brussels Sprouts:

Ingredients:

- ❖ 4 oz chicken thighs
- ❖ 1 cup Brussels sprouts, halved
- ❖ 1 tablespoon olive oil
- ❖ 1 teaspoon garlic powder
- ❖ Salt and pepper to taste

Preparation:

1. Preheat the oven to 425°F (220°C).
2. Rub chicken with olive oil, garlic powder, salt, and pepper.
3. Place chicken and Brussels sprouts on a baking sheet.
4. Bake until chicken is cooked through and Brussels sprouts are crispy.

Servings: 2

Nutritional Value: Calcium: 100mg, Vitamin D: 150 IU, Carbs: 10g, Fat: 15g

Cooking Time: 35 minutes

15. Vegetarian Lentil Soup:

Ingredients:

- ❖ 1 cup lentils, rinsed and drained
- ❖ 1/2 cup carrots, diced
- ❖ 1/2 cup celery, chopped
- ❖ 1/2 cup onions, diced
- ❖ 2 cloves garlic, minced
- ❖ 4 cups vegetable broth
- ❖ 1 teaspoon cumin
- ❖ 1/2 teaspoon turmeric
- ❖ Salt and pepper to taste

Preparation:

1. In a pot, sauté onions and garlic until fragrant.
2. Add lentils, carrots, celery, cumin, turmeric, salt, and pepper.
3. Pour in vegetable broth and simmer until lentils are tender.

Servings: 4   **Cooking Time:** 30 minutes

Nutritional Value: Calcium: 80mg, Vitamin D: 80 IU, Carbs: 40g, Fat: 2g

SNACK AND DESSERT RECIPES:

1. Banana Almond Smoothie:

Ingredients:

- ❖ 1 ripe banana
- ❖ 1 cup almond milk (unsweetened)
- ❖ 1 tablespoon almond butter
- ❖ Ice cubes (optional)

Preparation:

1. Blend banana, almond milk, and almond butter until smooth.
2. Add ice cubes if desired and blend again.
3. Pour into a glass and serve.

Servings: 1

Nutritional Value: Calcium: 200mg, Vitamin D: 30 IU, Carbs: 25g, Fat: 8g

Preparation Time: 5 minutes

2. Cottage Cheese with Pineapple:

Ingredients:

- ❖ 1/2 cup low-fat cottage cheese
- ❖ 1/2 cup fresh pineapple chunks
- ❖ 1 tablespoon shredded coconut

Preparation:

1. In a bowl, combine cottage cheese and pineapple.
2. Sprinkle shredded coconut on top.
3. Mix well and enjoy.

Servings: 1

Nutritional Value:

- ❖ Calcium: 180mg
- ❖ Vitamin D: 20 IU
- ❖ Carbs: 15g
- ❖ Fat: 5g

Preparation Time: 5 minutes

3. Roasted Chickpeas:

Ingredients:

- ❖ 1 can (15 oz) chickpeas, drained and rinsed
- ❖ 1 tablespoon olive oil
- ❖ 1 teaspoon smoked paprika
- ❖ 1/2 teaspoon garlic powder
- ❖ 1/2 teaspoon cumin
- ❖ Salt to taste

Preparation:

1. Preheat the oven to 400°F (200°C).
2. Pat dry chickpeas and place them on a baking sheet.
3. Drizzle with olive oil and sprinkle with smoked paprika, garlic powder, cumin, and salt.
4. Toss to coat evenly and roast for 20-25 minutes until crispy.
5. Allow to cool before serving.

Servings: 4   **Preparation Time:** 30 minutes

Nutritional Value: Calcium: 80mg, Vitamin D: 0 IU

Carbs: 15g, Fat: 4g

4. Baked Apple with Cinnamon:

Ingredients:

- ❖ 1 apple, cored and sliced
- ❖ 1/2 teaspoon cinnamon
- ❖ 1 tablespoon chopped walnuts
- ❖ 1 teaspoon honey

Preparation:

1. Preheat the oven to 375°F (190°C).
2. Place apple slices on a baking sheet.
3. Sprinkle with cinnamon and bake for 15-20 minutes until tender.
4. Remove from the oven, sprinkle with chopped walnuts, and drizzle with honey.
5. Serve warm.

Servings: 1

Nutritional Value: Calcium: 20mg, Vitamin D: 0 IU

Carbs: 25g, Fat: 3g

Preparation Time: 25 minutes

5. Chocolate Avocado Mousse:

Ingredients:

- ❖ 1 ripe avocado
- ❖ 2 tablespoons cocoa powder
- ❖ 2 tablespoons maple syrup
- ❖ 1/2 teaspoon vanilla extract

Preparation:

1. In a blender, combine avocado, cocoa powder, maple syrup, and vanilla extract.
2. Blend until smooth and creamy.
3. Refrigerate for 1-2 hours before serving.
4. Garnish with berries if desired.

Servings: 2

Nutritional Value:

- ❖ Calcium: 40mg
- ❖ Vitamin D: 0 IU
- ❖ Carbs: 15g
- ❖ Fat: 10g

Preparation Time: 10 minutes (+ chilling time)

6. Cucumber and Hummus Bites:

Ingredients:

- ❖ 1 cucumber, sliced
- ❖ 1/4 cup hummus (homemade or store-bought)
- ❖ Cherry tomatoes for topping

Preparation:

1. Slice cucumber into rounds.
2. Top each cucumber round with a small spoonful of hummus.
3. Place a cherry tomato on top of the hummus.
4. Serve chilled.

Servings: 4

Nutritional Value: Calcium: 40mg, Vitamin D: 0 IU, Carbs: 10g, Fat: 3g

Preparation Time: 10 minutes

7. Yogurt-Dipped Strawberries:

Ingredients:

- ❖ 1 cup strawberries, washed and dried
- ❖ 1/2 cup Greek yogurt (unsweetened)
- ❖ 1 tablespoon honey
- ❖ Preparation:
- ❖ In a bowl, mix Greek yogurt and honey.
- ❖ Dip each strawberry into the yogurt mixture, coating evenly.
- ❖ Place on a parchment-lined tray and freeze for 1-2 hours.
- ❖ Enjoy as a refreshing frozen treat.

Servings: 2

Nutritional Value:

- ❖ Calcium: 100mg
- ❖ Vitamin D: 0 IU
- ❖ Carbs: 20g
- ❖ Fat: 5g

Preparation Time: 15 minutes (+ freezing time)

JUICE AND SMOOTHIE RECIPES:

1. Green Calcium Boost Smoothie:

Ingredients:

- ❖ 1 cup kale, stems removed
- ❖ 1/2 cup low-fat yogurt
- ❖ 1/2 cup pineapple chunks
- ❖ 1/2 banana
- ❖ 1/2 cup almond milk (unsweetened)
- ❖ Ice cubes (optional)

Preparation:

1. Blend kale, yogurt, pineapple, banana, and almond milk until smooth.
2. Add ice cubes if desired and blend again.
3. Pour into a glass and enjoy.

Servings: 1

Nutritional Value: Calcium: 300mg, Vitamin D: 40 IU, Carbs: 30g, Fat: 8g

Preparation Time: 5 minutes

2. Berry Citrus Delight Juice:

Ingredients:

- ❖ 1/2 cup strawberries
- ❖ 1/2 cup blueberries
- ❖ 1/2 cup raspberries
- ❖ 1 orange, peeled and segmented
- ❖ 1/2 cup coconut water
- ❖ 1 teaspoon chia seeds

Preparation:

1. In a blender, combine strawberries, blueberries, raspberries, orange segments, coconut water, and chia seeds.
2. Blend until smooth.
3. Strain the mixture if a smoother juice is preferred.
4. Pour into a glass and serve.

Servings: 1

Nutritional Value: Calcium: 80mg, Vitamin D: 40 IU, Carbs: 25g, Fat: 2g

Preparation Time: 5 minutes

3. Tropical Bone Builder Smoothie:

Ingredients:

- ❖ 1/2 cup mango chunks
- ❖ 1/2 cup pineapple chunks
- ❖ 1/2 cup spinach
- ❖ 1/2 cup Greek yogurt
- ❖ 1/2 cup coconut milk (unsweetened)
- ❖ 1 tablespoon flaxseeds

Preparation:

1. Blend mango, pineapple, spinach, Greek yogurt, coconut milk, and flaxseeds until smooth.
2. Pour into a glass and serve immediately.

Servings: 1

Nutritional Value: Calcium: 250mg, Vitamin D: 30 IU, Carbs: 30g, Fat: 8g

Preparation Time: 5 minutes

4. Calcium-Rich Citrus Juice:

Ingredients:

- ❖ 2 oranges, peeled and segmented
- ❖ 1/2 grapefruit, peeled and segmented
- ❖ 1 kiwi, peeled and sliced
- ❖ 1 tablespoon honey
- ❖ 1/2 cup cold water

Preparation:

1. In a blender, combine orange segments, grapefruit segments, kiwi slices, honey, and cold water.
2. Blend until well combined.
3. Strain the mixture for a smoother juice, if desired.
4. Pour into a glass and serve over ice.

Servings: 1

Nutritional Value: Calcium: 100mg, Vitamin D: 20 IU, Carbs: 30g, Fat: 1g

Preparation Time: 5 minutes

5. Pomegranate Berry Bliss Smoothie:

Ingredients:

- ❖ 1/2 cup pomegranate seeds
- ❖ 1/2 cup mixed berries (strawberries, blueberries, raspberries)
- ❖ 1/2 cup plain yogurt
- ❖ 1/2 cup almond milk (unsweetened)
- ❖ 1 tablespoon pumpkin seeds

Preparation:

1. Blend pomegranate seeds, mixed berries, yogurt, almond milk, and pumpkin seeds until smooth.
2. Pour into a glass and serve.

Servings: 1

Nutritional Value: Calcium: 200mg, Vitamin D: 30 IU, Carbs: 30g, Fat: 7g

Preparation Time: 5 minutes

6. Avocado Spinach Power Juice:

Ingredients:

- ❖ 1/2 avocado, peeled and pitted
- ❖ 1 cup spinach
- ❖ 1 green apple, cored and sliced
- ❖ 1/2 cucumber, sliced
- ❖ 1/2 lemon, juiced
- ❖ 1 cup water

Preparation:

1. In a blender, combine avocado, spinach, green apple slices, cucumber slices, lemon juice, and water.
2. Blend until smooth.
3. Strain the mixture if desired.
4. Pour into a glass and serve.

Servings: 1

Nutritional Value: Calcium: 150mg, Vitamin D: 20 IU, Carbs: 20g, Fat: 8g

Preparation Time: 5 minutes

CONCLUSION

In concluding this **"Osteoporosis Diet Cookbook for Seniors,"** I am filled with gratitude for the opportunity to share a culinary journey that transcends the ordinary. As a nutritionist with a passion for promoting bone health, I've witnessed the transformative power of these delicious, calcium-rich recipes in the lives of many seniors facing the challenges of osteoporosis.

Within these pages, you've discovered not just a collection of meals, but a roadmap to stronger bones, vibrant health, and a life of vitality. The stories shared, the struggles overcome, and the triumphs celebrated are woven into the very fabric of this cookbook. It's a testament to the resilience of the human spirit and the unwavering belief that, even in the face of osteoporosis, one can cultivate a life rich in flavor and fulfillment.

As you embark on this journey, remember that each recipe is a gesture of care and a promise of nourishment for your bones and overall well-being. The scientifically proven ingredients are not just culinary elements; they are the building blocks of resilience, strength, and joy.

I invite you to adopt this osteoporosis-friendly diet not just as a regimen but as a celebration of your commitment to a life well-lived. Let every bite be a declaration of self-love and an investment in your health. Embrace these recipes not merely as sustenance but as a daily ritual of empowerment.

May your journey be filled with the savor of good health, the joy of rediscovered strength, and the promise of a future where osteoporosis is met with resilience and delicious defiance. You have the power to shape your story, and this cookbook is your ally on the path to a life brimming with vitality.

Here's to strong bones, radiant health, and the delectable joy of living well!

WEEKLY MEAL JOURNAL

WEEK _____   MONTH _____

MONDAY

SATURDAY

TUESDAY

SUNDAY

WEDNESDAY

SHOPPING LIST

- ○ _____
- ○ _____
- ○ _____
- ○ _____
- ○ _____
- ○ _____
- ○ _____
- ○ _____

THURSDAY

FRIDAY

NOTES:
- ○ _____
- ○ _____
- ○ _____
- ○ _____

WEEKLY MEAL JOURNAL

WEEK _____   MONTH _____

MONDAY

SATURDAY

TUESDAY

SUNDAY

WEDNESDAY

SHOPPING LIST

○ _____
○ _____
○ _____
○ _____
○ _____
○ _____
○ _____
○ _____

THURSDAY

FRIDAY

○ NOTES:
○ _____
○ _____
○ _____

WEEKLY MEAL JOURNAL

WEEK _____   MONTH _____

MONDAY	SATURDAY

TUESDAY	SUNDAY

WEDNESDAY

SHOPPING LIST
- ○ _____
- ○ _____
- ○ _____
- ○ _____
- ○ _____
- ○ _____
- ○ _____
- ○ _____

THURSDAY

FRIDAY

NOTES:
- ○ _____
- ○ _____
- ○ _____
- ○ _____

WEEKLY MEAL JOURNAL

WEEK _____ MONTH _____

MONDAY

SATURDAY

TUESDAY

SUNDAY

WEDNESDAY

SHOPPING LIST

- ○ _____
- ○ _____
- ○ _____
- ○ _____
- ○ _____
- ○ _____
- ○ _____
- ○ _____

THURSDAY

FRIDAY

NOTES:
- ○ _____
- ○ _____
- ○ _____
- ○ _____

WEEKLY MEAL JOURNAL

WEEK _____   MONTH _____

MONDAY

SATURDAY

TUESDAY

SUNDAY

WEDNESDAY

SHOPPING LIST

○ _____
○ _____
○ _____
○ _____
○ _____
○ _____
○ _____
○ _____

THURSDAY

FRIDAY

NOTES:

○ _____
○ _____
○ _____
○ _____

WEEKLY MEAL JOURNAL

WEEK _____   MONTH _____

MONDAY

SATURDAY

TUESDAY

SUNDAY

WEDNESDAY

SHOPPING LIST

- ○ _____
- ○ _____
- ○ _____
- ○ _____
- ○ _____
- ○ _____
- ○ _____
- ○ _____

THURSDAY

FRIDAY

NOTES:

- ○ _____
- ○ _____
- ○ _____
- ○ _____

WEEKLY MEAL JOURNAL

WEEK _____ MONTH _____

MONDAY

SATURDAY

TUESDAY

SUNDAY

WEDNESDAY

SHOPPING LIST

○ _____
○ _____
○ _____
○ _____
○ _____
○ _____
○ _____
○ _____

THURSDAY

FRIDAY

NOTES:

○ _____
○ _____
○ _____
○ _____

WEEKLY MEAL JOURNAL

WEEK _____   MONTH _____

MONDAY

SATURDAY

TUESDAY

SUNDAY

WEDNESDAY

SHOPPING LIST

- ○ _____
- ○ _____
- ○ _____
- ○ _____
- ○ _____
- ○ _____
- ○ _____
- ○ _____

THURSDAY

FRIDAY

NOTES:
- ○ _____
- ○ _____
- ○ _____
- ○ _____

WEEKLY MEAL JOURNAL

WEEK _____   MONTH _____

| MONDAY | SATURDAY |

| TUESDAY | SUNDAY |

| WEDNESDAY | SHOPPING LIST |

○ _____
○ _____
○ _____
○ _____

| THURSDAY |

○ _____
○ _____
○ _____
○ _____

| FRIDAY | NOTES: |

○ _____
○ _____
○ _____
○ _____

WEEKLY MEAL JOURNAL

WEEK _____   MONTH _____

MONDAY

SATURDAY

TUESDAY

SUNDAY

WEDNESDAY

SHOPPING LIST

- ○ _____
- ○ _____
- ○ _____
- ○ _____
- ○ _____
- ○ _____
- ○ _____
- ○ _____
- ○ _____

THURSDAY

FRIDAY

NOTES:

- ○ _____
- ○ _____
- ○ _____
- ○ _____

WEEKLY MEAL JOURNAL

WEEK ————————— MONTH —————————

MONDAY

TUESDAY

WEDNESDAY

THURSDAY

FRIDAY

SATURDAY

SUNDAY

SHOPPING LIST
- ○ _____
- ○ _____
- ○ _____
- ○ _____
- ○ _____
- ○ _____
- ○ _____
- ○ _____

NOTES:
- ○ _____
- ○ _____
- ○ _____
- ○ _____

WEEKLY MEAL JOURNAL

WEEK _____   MONTH _____

MONDAY

SATURDAY

TUESDAY

SUNDAY

WEDNESDAY

SHOPPING LIST
- ○ _____
- ○ _____
- ○ _____
- ○ _____
- ○ _____
- ○ _____
- ○ _____
- ○ _____

THURSDAY

FRIDAY

NOTES:
- ○ _____
- ○ _____
- ○ _____
- ○ _____

WEEKLY MEAL JOURNAL

WEEK _____   MONTH _____

MONDAY		SATURDAY

TUESDAY		SUNDAY

WEDNESDAY

SHOPPING LIST
- ○ _____
- ○ _____
- ○ _____
- ○ _____
- ○ _____
- ○ _____
- ○ _____
- ○ _____
- ○ _____

THURSDAY

FRIDAY

NOTES:
- ○ _____
- ○ _____
- ○ _____
- ○ _____

Made in the USA
Columbia, SC
20 January 2024

30718801R00065